HOW TO BE A GERMOPHOBE

Avoiding Sickness In Today's Germy World

By

Pam June

authorHOUSE®

AuthorHouse™
1663 Liberty Drive
Bloomington, IN 47403
www.authorhouse.com
Phone: 1-800-839-8640

First published by AuthorHouse 9/3/2009

ISBN: 978-1-4490-2060-6 (e)
ISBN: 978-1-4490-2059-0 (sc)

Library of Congress Control Number: 2009909027

Printed in the United States of America
Bloomington, Indiana

This book is printed on acid-free paper.

FOREWORD

You know the old saying "an ounce of prevention is worth a pound of cure." This book is intended to be an "ounce of prevention." It is not based on scientific research or studies. It's about being careful to avoid as many illness-causing germs as possible and protecting yourself and others against potentially becoming sick. The reality is that there are a lot of scary germs out there. The most recent one is H1N1, or swine flu. I have personally experienced a "pound of cure" in the form of MRSA (methicillin resistant staphylococcus aureus). It was a nightmare that could have been prevented and it is one of the main reasons I have become a germophobe. I also hate getting sick, especially colds, so I am extra careful to keep my hands clean and stay away from sick people. I have taught my kids the same, but, occasionally, they bring colds home from school or church anyway. That is where immunity-boosting supplements come in handy. I swear by them, especially in the wintertime. You can't avoid all germs; they are a part of life. Just be careful and try to avoid as many as you can.

Public bathrooms

Most public bathrooms are basically disgusting and dirty. If you need to sit on the toilet, line the seat very well with paper. And, of course, always flush with your foot or a piece of toilet paper. Never touch the handle with your bare hand.

While automatic faucets are great, not all bathrooms have them. Use a paper towel to turn the water on and get some soap, and then throw it away. Get another paper towel ready to grab so you can dry your hands with it. Wash your hands thoroughly for about sixty seconds, or the time it takes to sing the alphabet song in your head. Leave the water on until you dry your hands. Use your paper towel to turn the water off and also open the door with it. Touching the faucet with your bare hands will transfer germs back to your hands. If the bathroom only has hand dryers, use some toilet paper instead for the faucets, soap dispenser, and door. If you happen across a bathroom that has no soap, always keep a supply of hand sanitizer or sanitizing hand wipes in your car or purse.

Avoid putting your purse or any other items on the floor. If there is absolutely no place to hang your purse and you have to put it down, put a couple of clean paper towels under it.

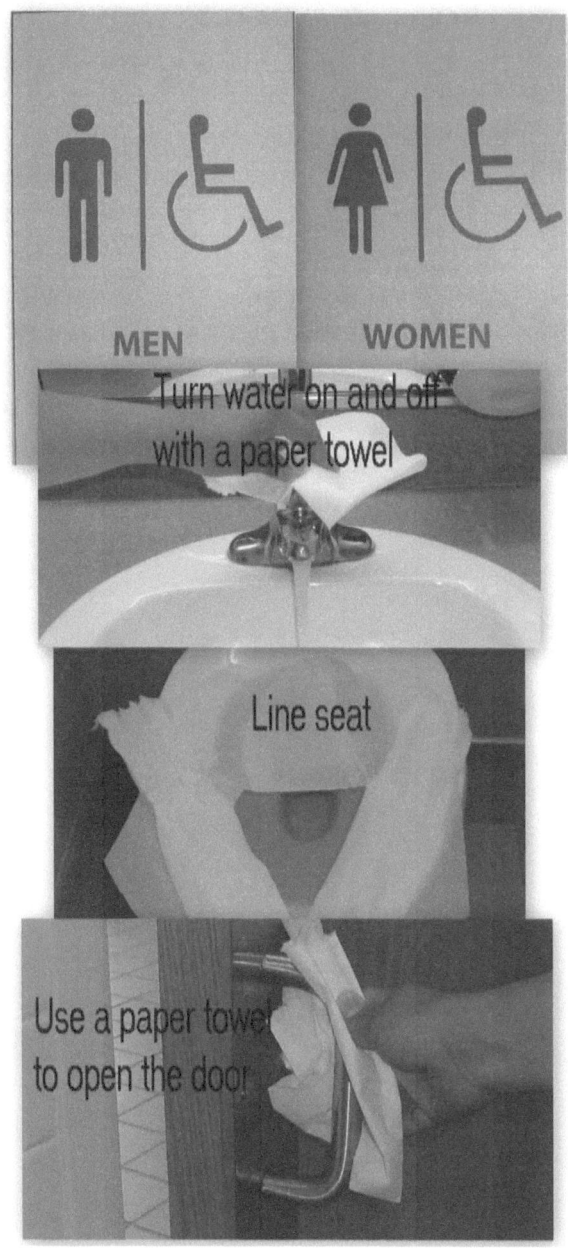

MEN   WOMEN

Turn water on and off with a paper towel

Line seat

Use a paper towel to open the door

Diaper Changing Stations
In Public Bathrooms

Do your best to avoid public diaper changing stations. If you have a stroller with you, use that. If you can sit somewhere and put the baby on your lap, do that, unless the child is too big. Another option is to go outside and change the baby in the car. If there is no practical alternative, wipe the surface of the changing table with a sanitizing wipe, cover it with paper towels, then put a changing pad over the paper towels. Of course, don't forget to wash your own hands after changing a diaper.

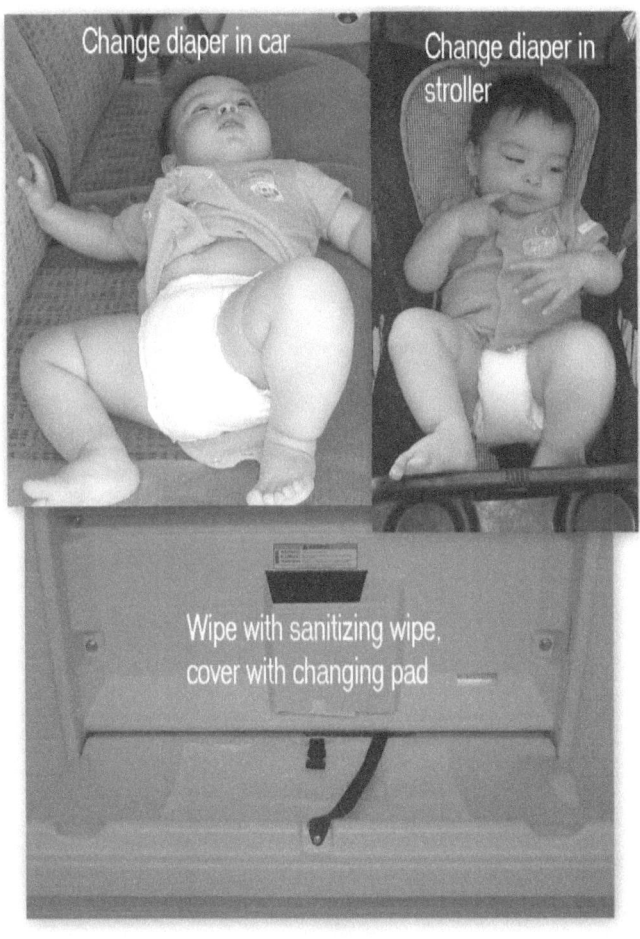

DRINKING FOUNTAINS

If at all possible, avoid the drinking fountain. They get a lot of backwash from a lot of people and, generally, are not sanitized. Carry a water bottle with you instead. If you absolutely must drink from a fountain, let the water run a little while first. As a back up, take an immunity-boosting supplement as soon as possible after drinking from a fountain.

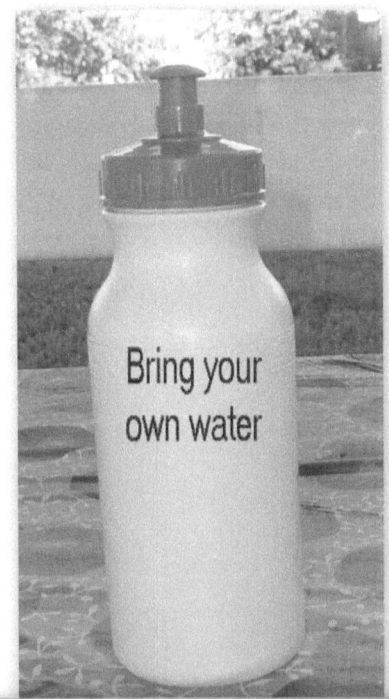

Bring your
own water

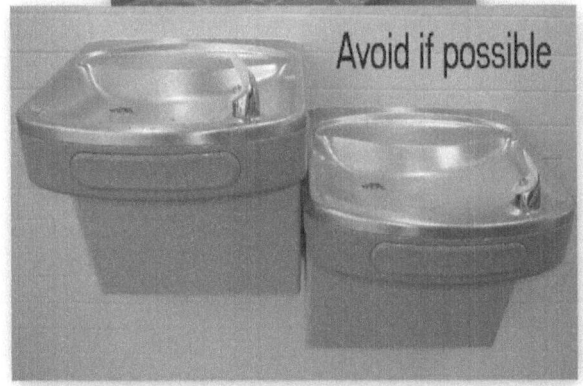

Avoid if possible

OPENING DOORS

Automatic doors are wonderful but they are not everywhere. If there is a handicap door button available that opens the door, push that with your knee or elbow to avoid touching the door handle. If the door opens in, push it with your back. If it opens out, keep a tissue or napkin in your pocket to open the door with and then throw it away. Another trick is to put your car key over your finger and use it to open the door. The keys will need to be cleaned periodically but the point is to keep your hands clean. If you have no choice but to touch the door, try to pick a spot that is less likely to be used as much and sanitize your hands afterwards.

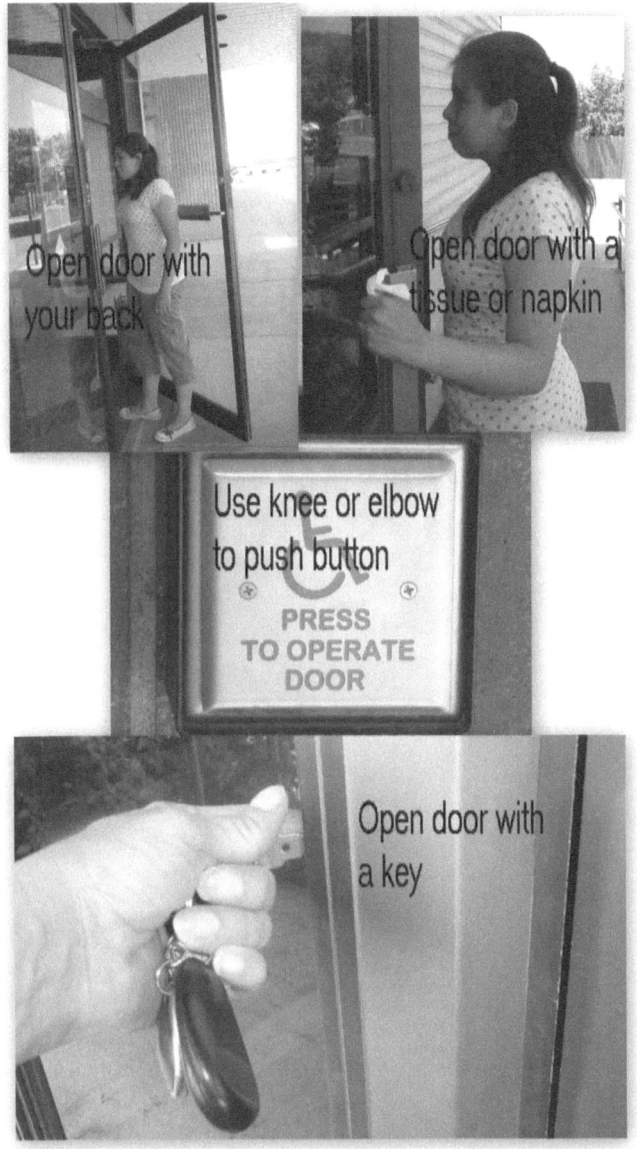

FAST FOOD RESTAURANTS
AND FOOD COURTS

When eating fast food, first of all take a look at the food preparation area if you can see it. Watch for sanitary practices like using gloves and hand washing. If it seems dirty or unsanitary, pass and go somewhere else. If you have a supply of sanitizing wipes with you, use one to wipe off the tabletop. If not, keep your food on the tray or on top of the wrappers. If you are sitting at a table instead of a booth, use your foot to pull the chair out. Avoid play areas in fast food restaurants. Eating combined with playing on public play equipment is a good way to get sick.

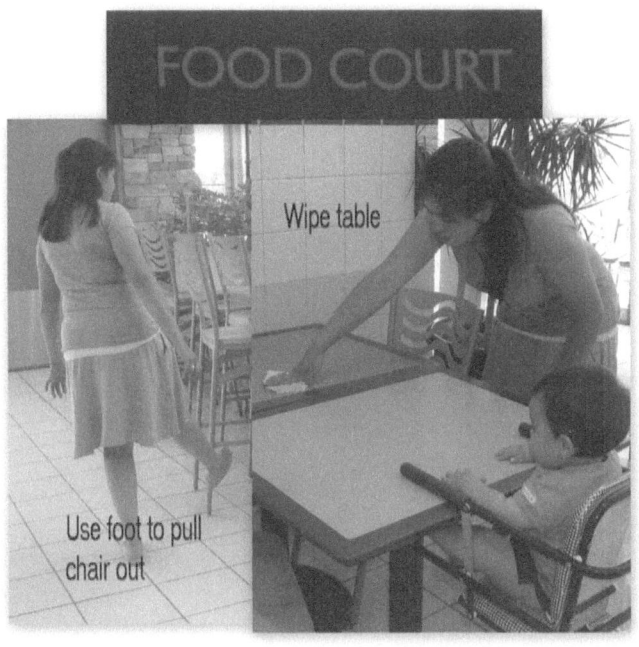

ALL YOU CAN EAT BUFFET RESTAURANTS

Be aware that there is a higher risk of food poisoning from this type of restaurant. These restaurants are usually crowded so a lot of people are touching the utensils. Keep a supply of hand sanitizer or wipes on your table. Wipe your hands every time you serve food at the buffet line. If the food looks like it has been sitting out too long, pass on that item.

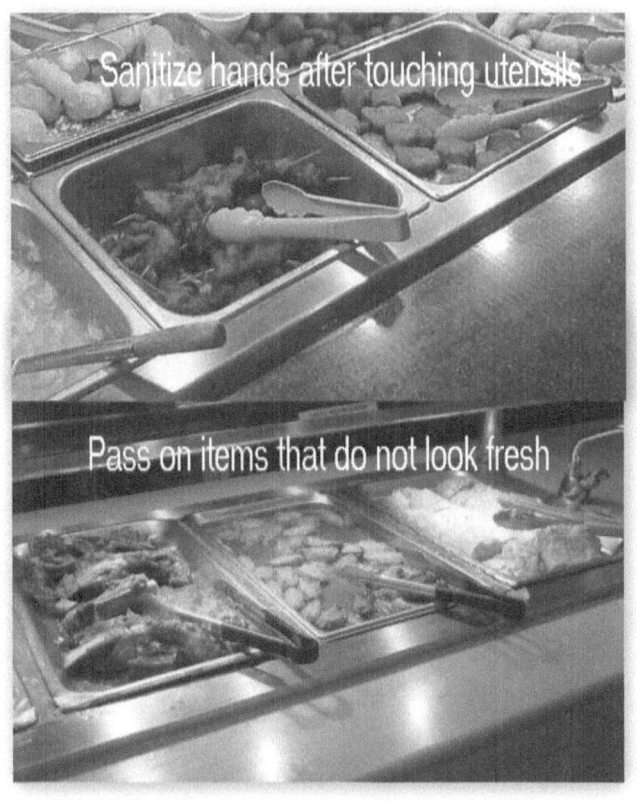

SELF SERVE FOUNTAIN DRINKS

Most fast food restaurants, buffet restaurants, and convenience stores have self serve fountain drinks. You want to keep your fingertips clean so you don't transfer germs from your fingers onto the straw. You can grab a napkin and use that to press the button or use your knuckle to press the button. If possible, use your own cup and lid. You don't know how many hands have touched the cups and lids that are provided.

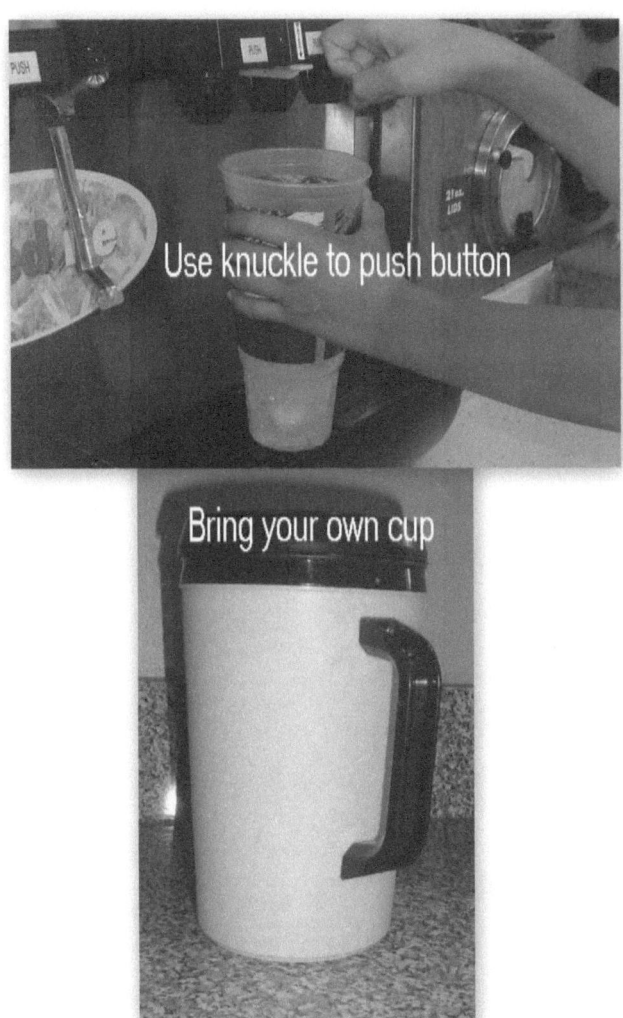

RESTAURANT HIGH CHAIRS

If you have a young child that requires a high chair, your best bet is to bring your own or use a seat cover. There are portable high chairs that fold up for storage and clip to a table for use (the table should be wiped off before the seat is attached). There are also seat covers that work in restaurant high chairs and grocery carts. They cover the entire surface of the seat to prevent kids from touching them. If you don't have your own portable high chair or seat cover, be sure to sanitize the seats that are provided.

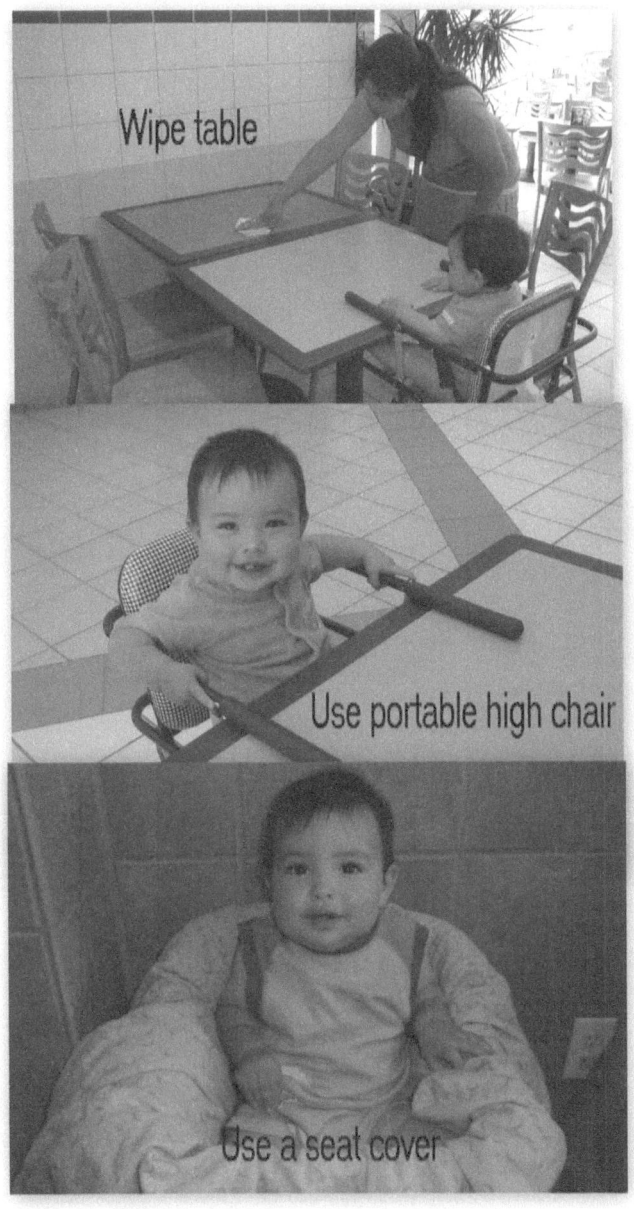

DINING RESTAURANTS

When dining out, be observant of the overall cleanliness of the restaurant. Sanitize your hands after handling the menu. Pass on the ice in your drink, unless you are sure it is not coming into contact with anybody's hands in any way. The ice scoop should be stored in a clean place outside of the ice machine so the handle never touches the ice. Otherwise, germs from hands that may be handling money and other things are put directly into the ice. Make sure ground meat is thoroughly cooked to avoid food poisoning due to e-coli. Make sure eggs are well done to avoid salmonella poisoning.

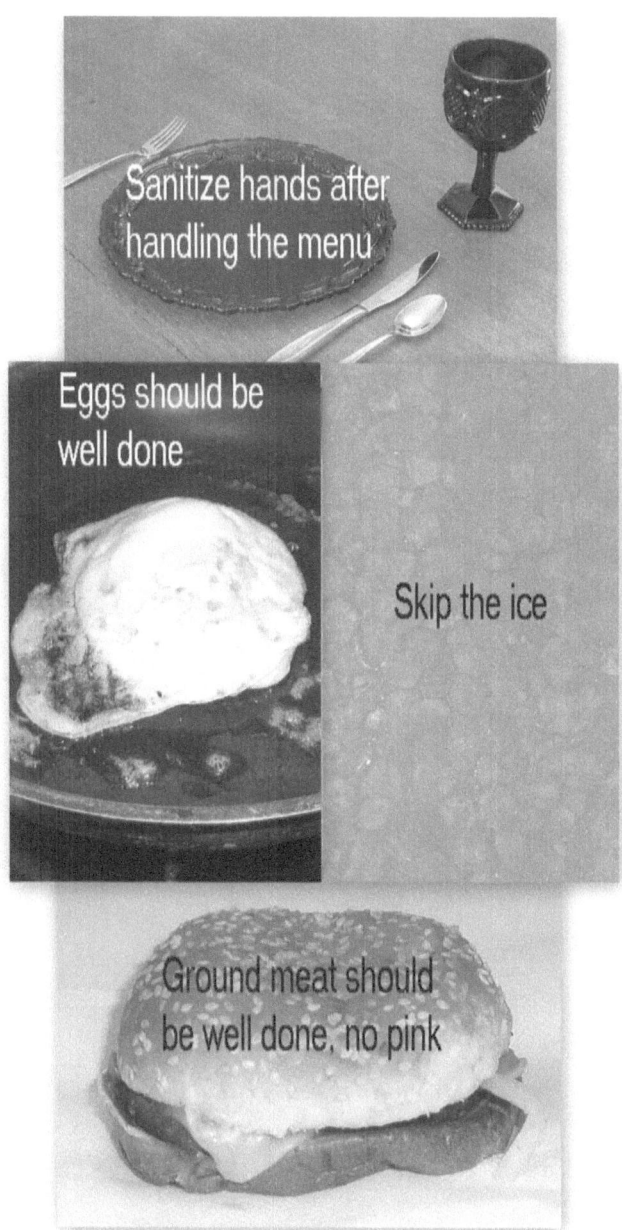

Sanitize hands after handling the menu

Eggs should be well done

Skip the ice

Ground meat should be well done, no pink

Grocery Carts

Most stores have sanitizing wipes near the carts now. Take advantage of them and wipe off the cart handle before you touch it. If the store does not have sanitizing wipes available, keep a supply of your own handy. If you have small children, there are seat covers available to purchase that cover the entire seat and have their own seatbelt. This prevents children from touching or sucking on the cart. While the carts designed to look like trucks or racecars are cute, they are also full of germs. It is best to just avoid them. If you do use one, wipe off all surfaces that a child might touch and sanitize the child's hands when you are done with it. Don't allow children to put their mouths on the any part of a grocery cart, including the seatbelt.

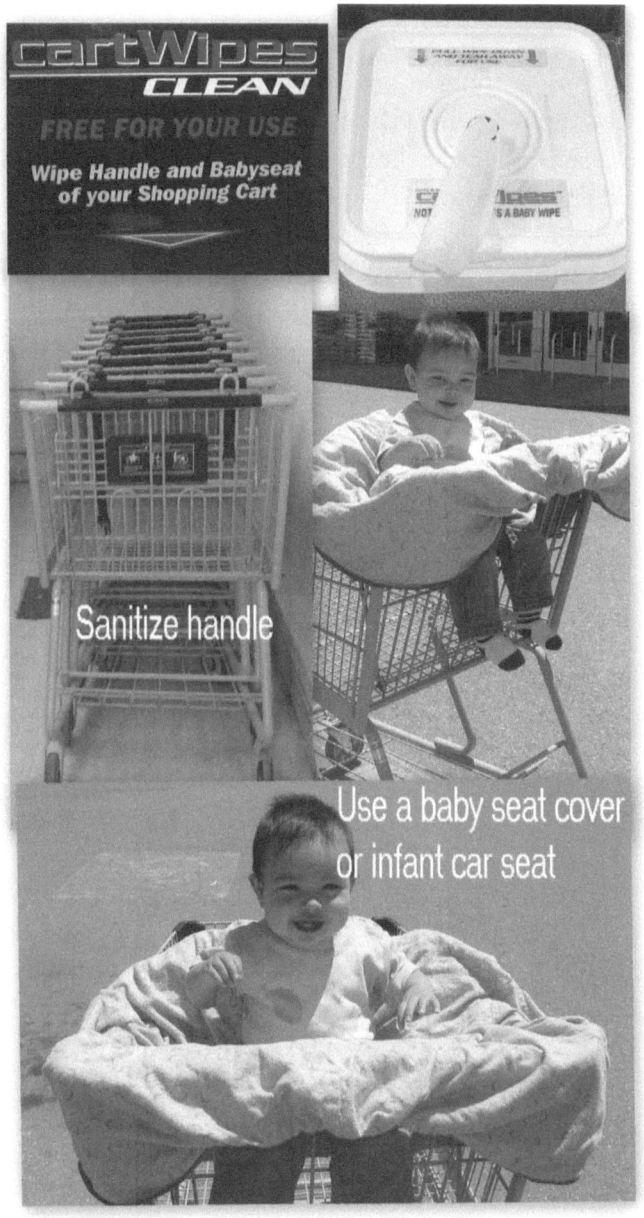

SELF-CHECKOUTS

There is nothing more annoying than a sick cashier that coughs on their hands and then touches all of your purchases. Self-checkouts are great, especially during cold and flu season. It's still a good idea to sanitize your hands after you touch the self-checkout terminal. If self-checkouts are not available and you end up in a line where the cashier is obviously sick, don't be afraid to switch to another line. It's better to wait a little longer than it is to end up getting sick.

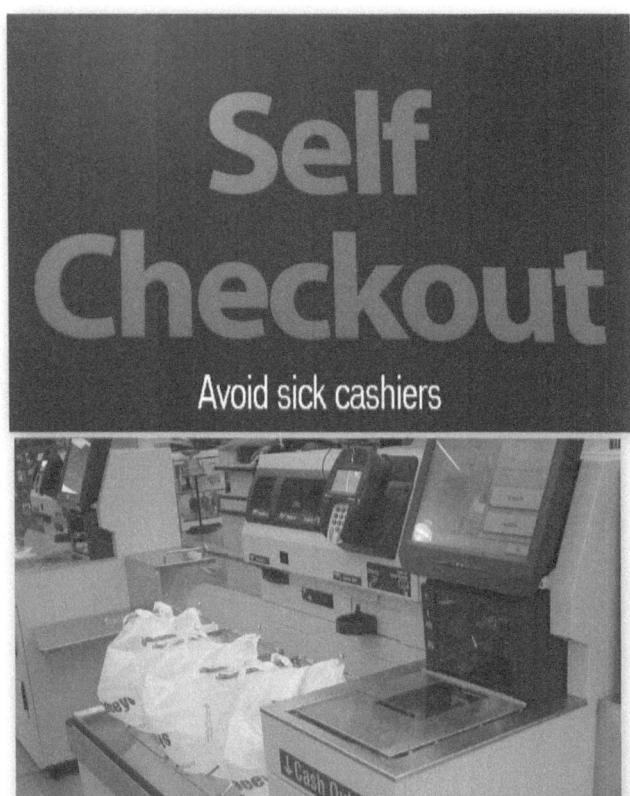

Using Credit/Debit Cards

Keep a pen of your own handy when paying with a credit card so you don't have to borrow one to sign the receipt. You never know how many people may have touched it. If you are using a credit/debit card machine, push the buttons with the corner of your card or your knuckles. If you have to touch the pen or buttons on the machine, sanitize your hands afterwards.

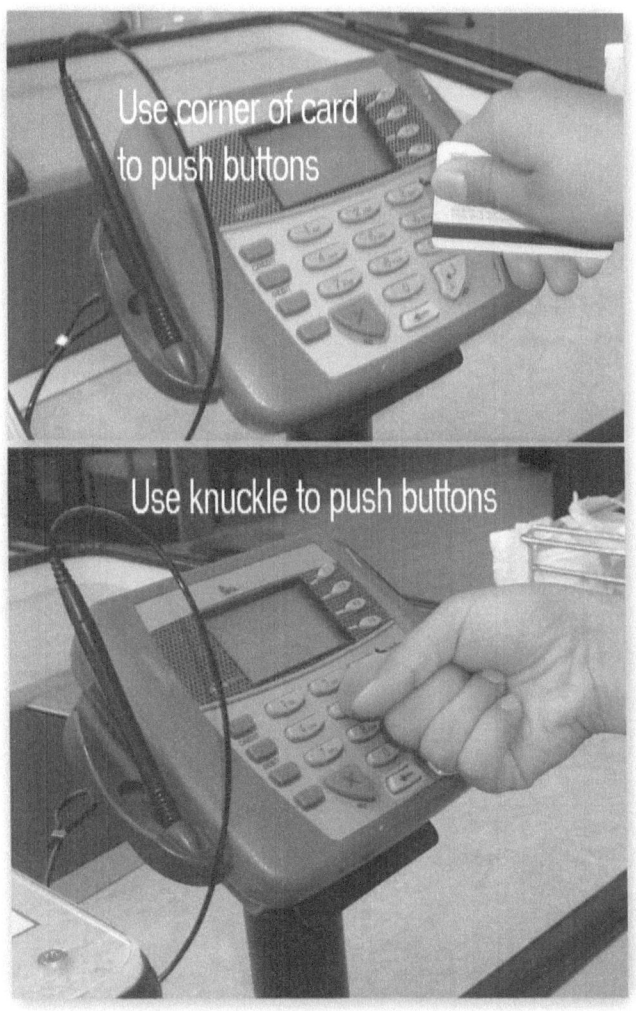

Use corner of card to push buttons

Use knuckle to push buttons

Automatic Teller Machines

At the ATM, use a tissue or napkin, if you have one, to push the buttons. If you must touch the buttons with your hands, use your knuckles to avoid getting germs on your fingertips. Sanitize your hands when you are done. It's not a bad idea to sanitize your hands after handling money anyway.

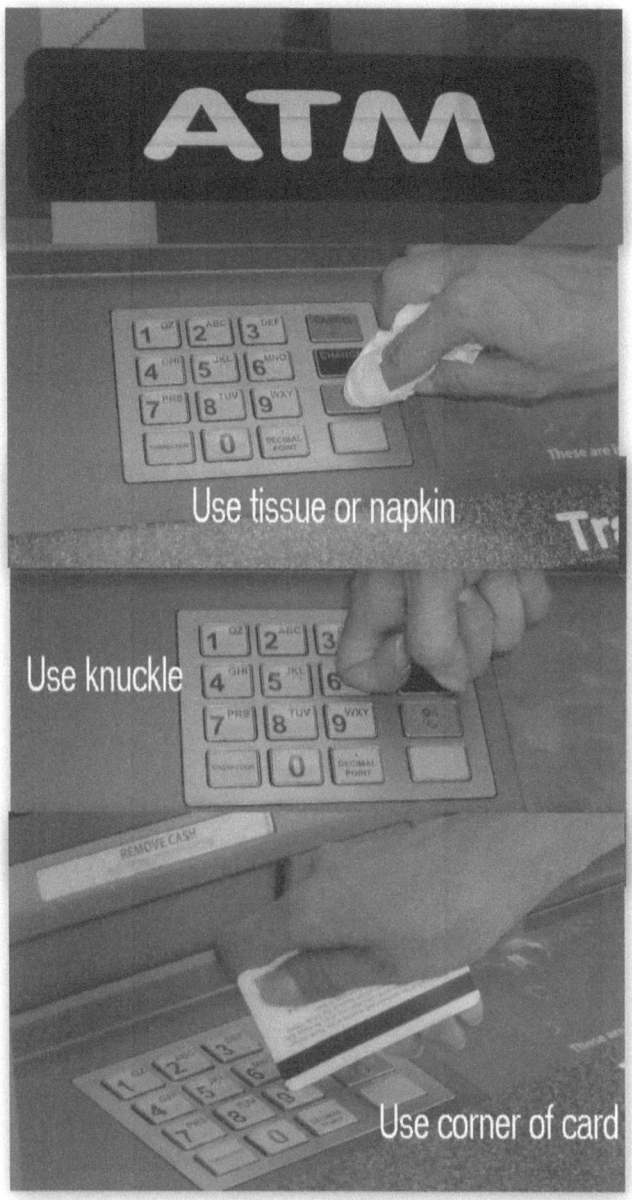

Gas Pumps

When pumping gas, get a paper towel if there are any available and use it to press the buttons and hold the handle of the gas pump. If there are no paper towels available, sanitize your hands when you are done. If you get gas on your hands, use hand wipes instead of hand sanitizer so the gas gets wiped off.

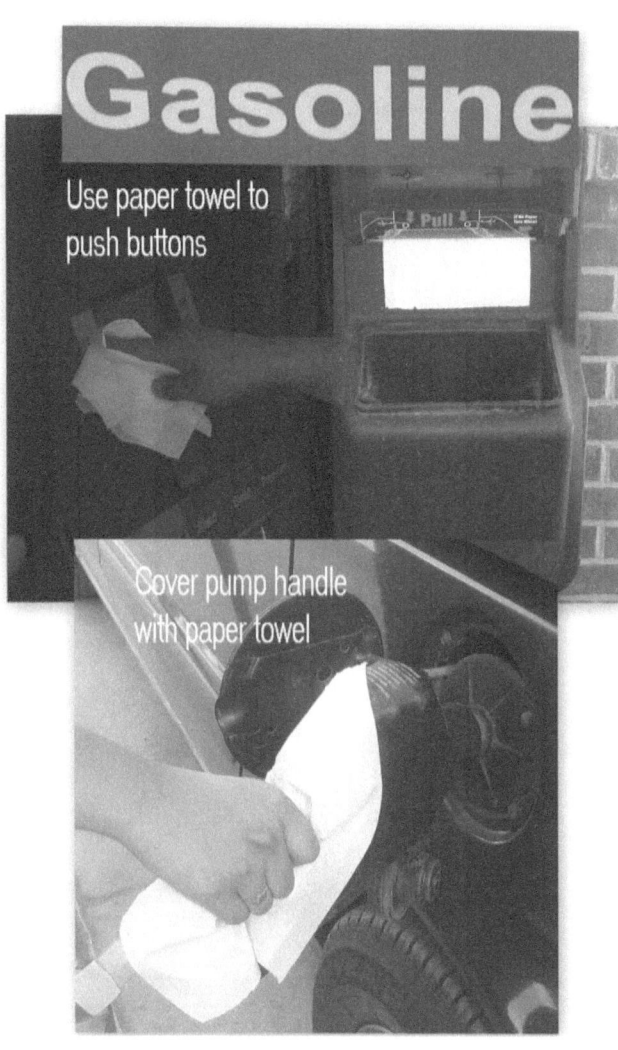

Gasoline

Use paper towel to push buttons

Cover pump handle with paper towel

HOLIDAY SHOPPING

Since the Christmas holiday season is during the height of cold and flu season, there are always people coughing everywhere you go. The stores are also more crowded, which makes it harder to keep your distance. Your best bet is to take an immunity-boosting supplement before you go out and avoid touching things as much as possible. Also, sanitize your hands often.

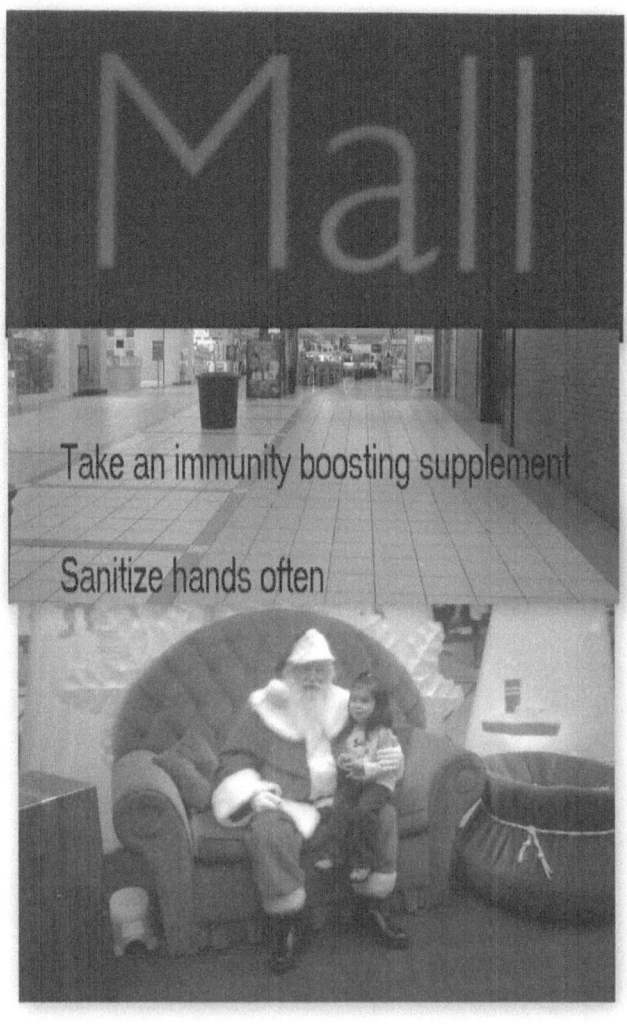

ELEVATORS

Press all elevator buttons with your elbow, wrist, or knuckle to avoid getting germs on your fingertips and spreading them. Avoid getting on an elevator with people who are obviously sick. Since germs can linger in the air for a while, it might be safer to take the stairs if you are able to, especially if you observe someone coughing as they go in or come out.

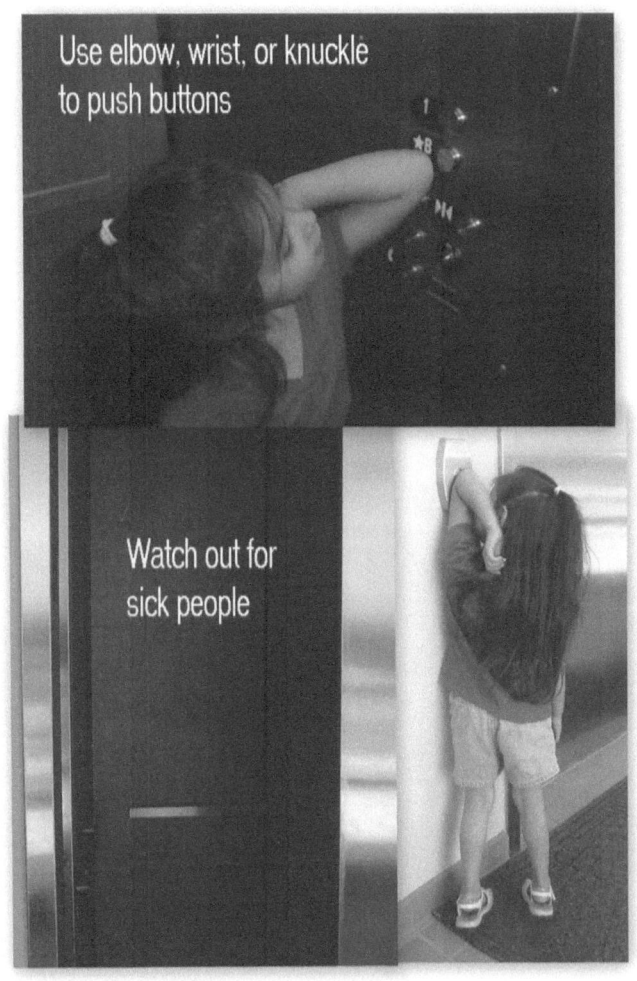

Use elbow, wrist, or knuckle to push buttons

Watch out for sick people

ESCALATORS/STAIRS

When riding on an escalator, if you have good balance, avoid touching the handrail altogether. Assist small children so they don't have to touch the handrail. If you must use the handrail, either use a tissue to cover it or be sure to sanitize your hands afterwards. The same applies to stairways.

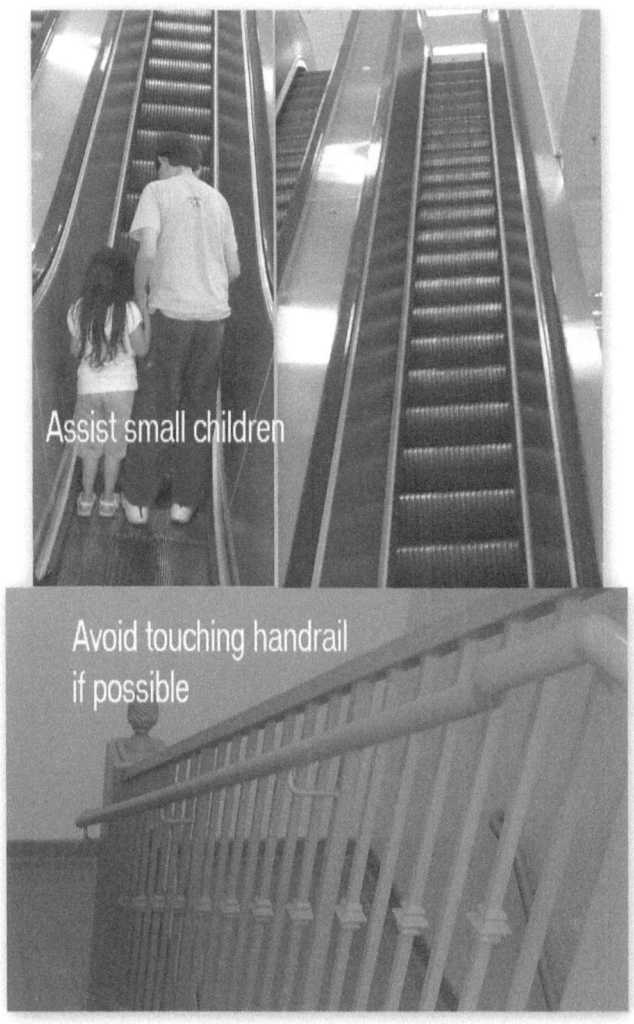

Assist small children

Avoid touching handrail
if possible

FRESH PRODUCE

With all of the breakouts of salmonella and e-coli
contamination related to produce items, it can be scary
to buy fresh fruit and vegetables. Try to buy locally
grown produce as much a possible. Be sure to wash
everything thoroughly. If it is something that will be
cooked, be sure to cook it thoroughly. If you have the
space for a garden, grow as much of your own produce
as possible.

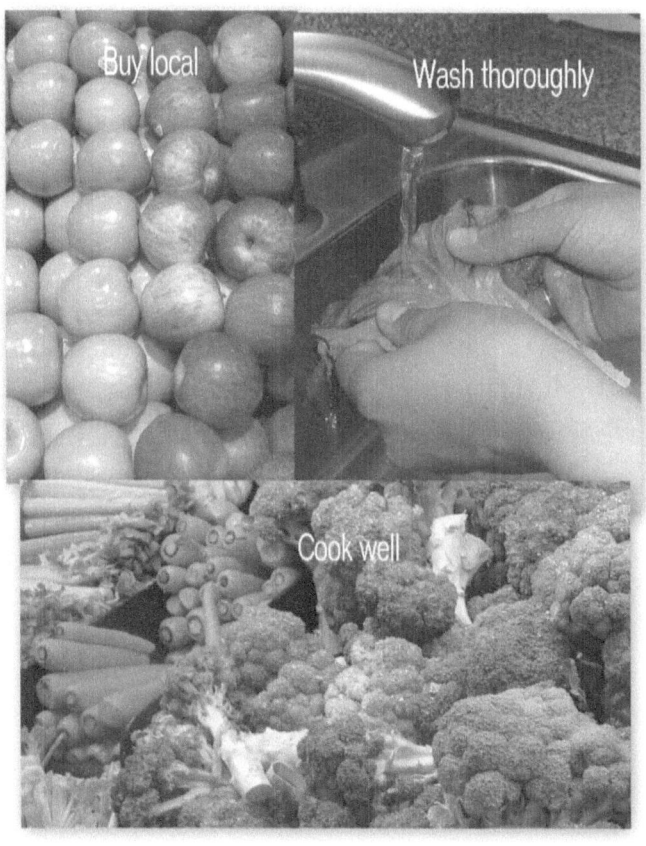

HANDLING RAW MEAT

When purchasing meat at the store, use the plastic bags that are provided to pick the meat package up. Put your hand inside the bag and pick the meat up with that hand. Pull the bag up around the meat. This prevents germs from getting on your hands and the bag prevents the meat from leaking on other items.

It is best to wear disposable rubber gloves to handle raw meat. This prevents germs from getting trapped under your fingernails and spread to other things. Sanitize all surfaces that raw meat may have come in contact with. Never use a wooden cutting board for raw meat. Use a plastic one that is dishwasher safe. Don't touch any other surfaces such as door handles or drawers until you have removed the gloves and washed your hands. If you do not have rubber gloves available, be sure to wash your hands thoroughly at least twice and don't forget to scrub under your fingernails. Also, make sure all meat, especially ground meat, is thoroughly cooked.

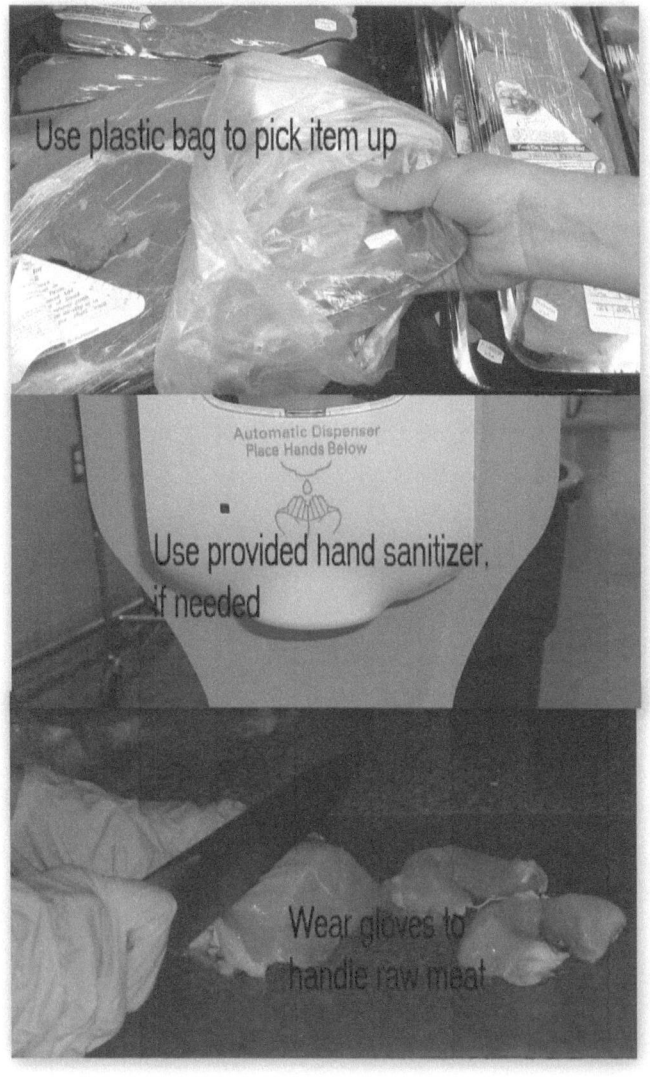

HANDLING RAW EGGS

When purchasing eggs, use the same method as purchasing meat. Stores don't usually have plastic bags near the egg section, so you will need to pick up an extra one in the produce section or the meat aisle. Put your hand inside the bag and use it to open the carton and check for broken eggs. If there are no broken eggs, pick it up and pull the bag up over the carton.

It probably isn't necessary to wear rubber gloves to crack open an egg. Washing your hands thoroughly after handling raw eggs is sufficient. Clean up any drips or spills with sanitizing cleaner.

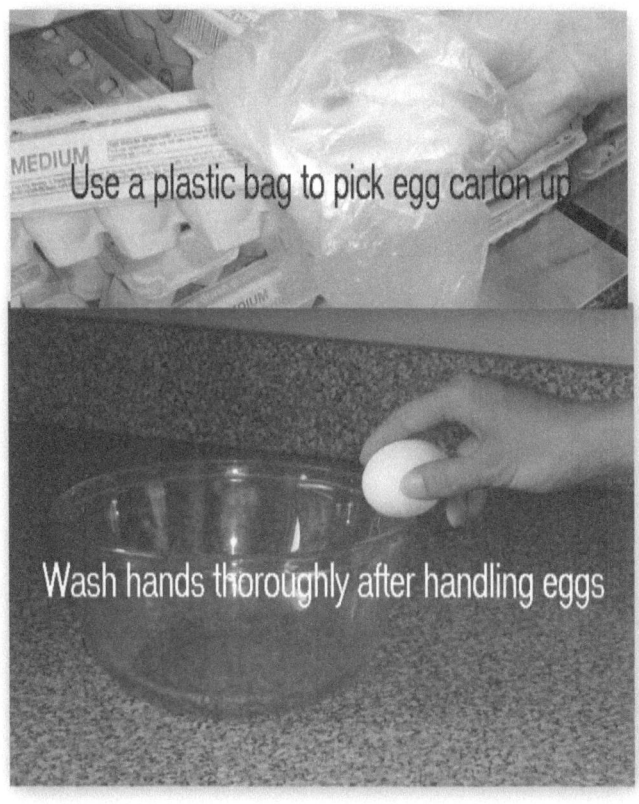

Use a plastic bag to pick egg carton up

Wash hands thoroughly after handling eggs

BAKING

Many recipes, especially cookies, contain raw eggs. Years ago, it was fun and delicious to eat raw cookie dough, but now, the risk of salmonella is not worth it. Avoid any raw dough that contains eggs and bake well. If you really need a treat and you can't wait for the baking time, grab a handful of chocolate chips before they are put into the batter. Be sure to wash your hands thoroughly after handling raw eggs and dough. Make sure the surface that the baked goods will be set on to cool is also sanitized. Never wipe the counters with a sponge! Use a clean dishrag instead.

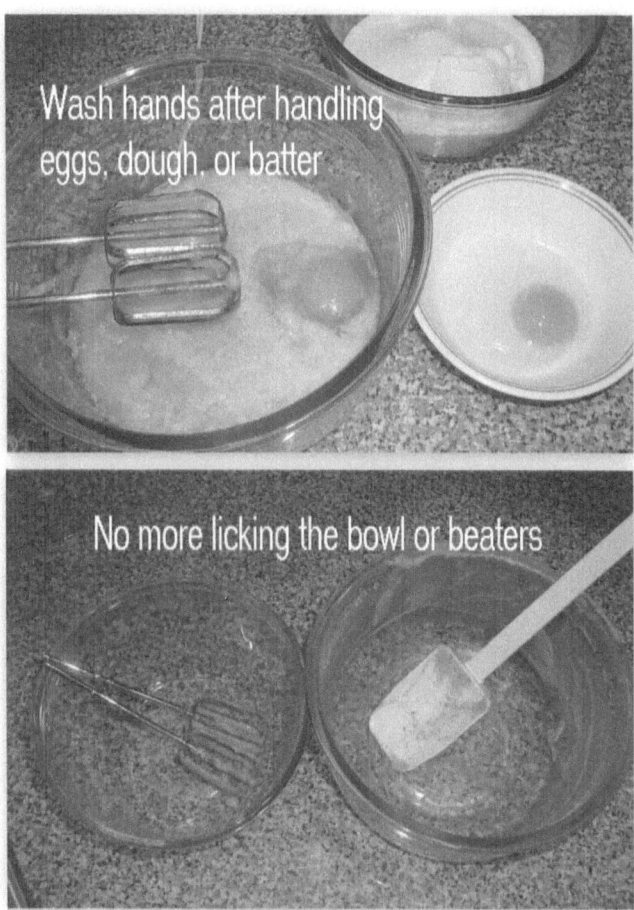

Wash hands after handling eggs, dough, or batter

No more licking the bowl or beaters

LIBRARY BOOKS

Your local library is a great resource. There are summer reading programs, story time for children, homework helps, and some great books to read. There is no need to miss out on the benefits of a library as long as you are careful. Obviously, you can't sanitize every page of the books you check out, but, as a precaution, you can wipe off the cover and binding with a sanitizing wipe. Don't forget to sanitize your hands after handling library books.

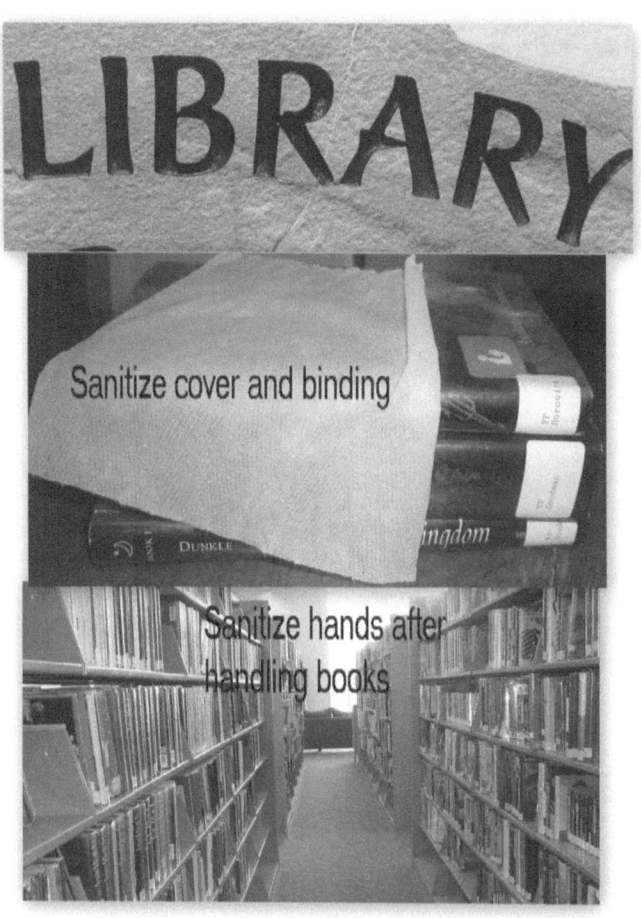

Movie Rentals

Like the pages of library books, you can't sanitize a DVD without ruining it, but you can wipe off the case with a sanitizing wipe. Don't forget to sanitize your hands when you leave the video store.

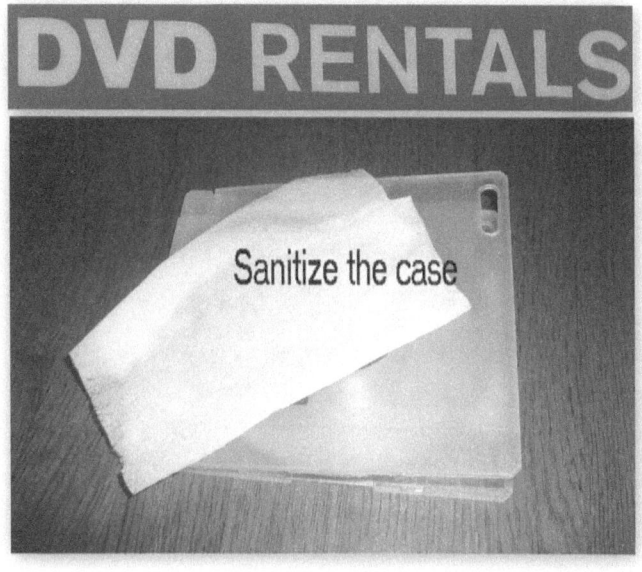

THRIFT STORES/YARD SALES

For those who love bargain and treasure hunting, don't let a fear of germs stop you. Just be sure to sanitize everything you have purchased secondhand. Clothing, small stuffed animals, linens, and etc. can be thrown in the washing machine. The dishwasher is also a great way to sanitize anything that is dishwasher safe, including plastic toys or other non-dish items. Upholstery cleaners can be used on big-ticket items such as sofas or mattresses, although it is better to pass on anything that is heavily soiled. Use your best judgment.

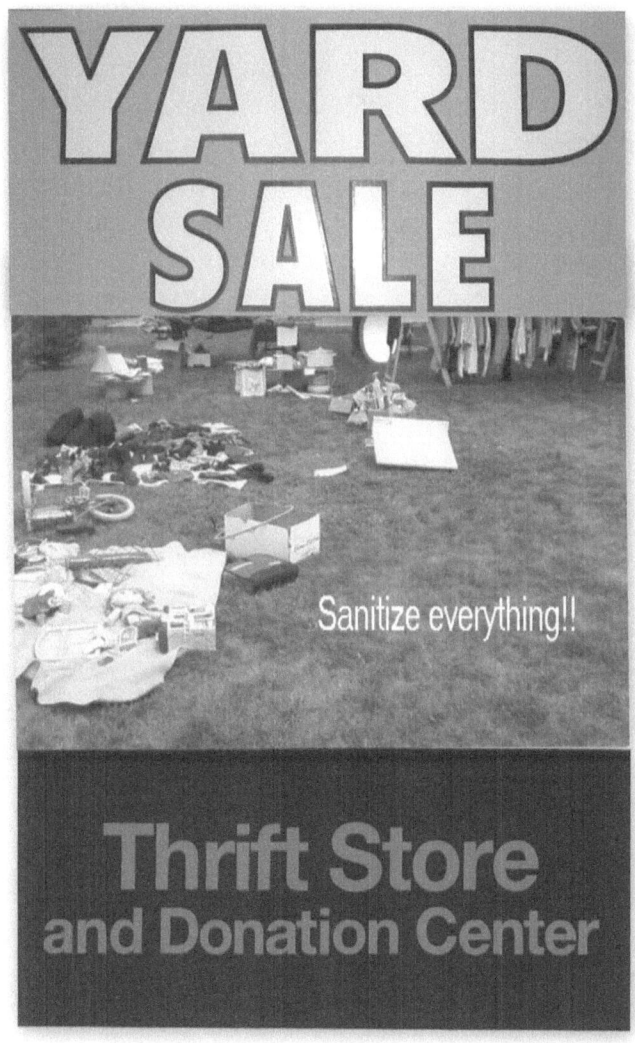

School

If you have kids in school, especially elementary school, there are germs everywhere. If it is allowed, send a water bottle with your child and tell them to avoid the drinking fountain. Teach them good hand washing practices. Send hand sanitizer or sanitizing hand wipes in their backpacks and lunches. Teach them to always wash their hands before eating at school. Tell them to stay as far away as possible from other kids who are sick. If you have the time and are able to, volunteer to go in and sanitize the classroom once in a while.

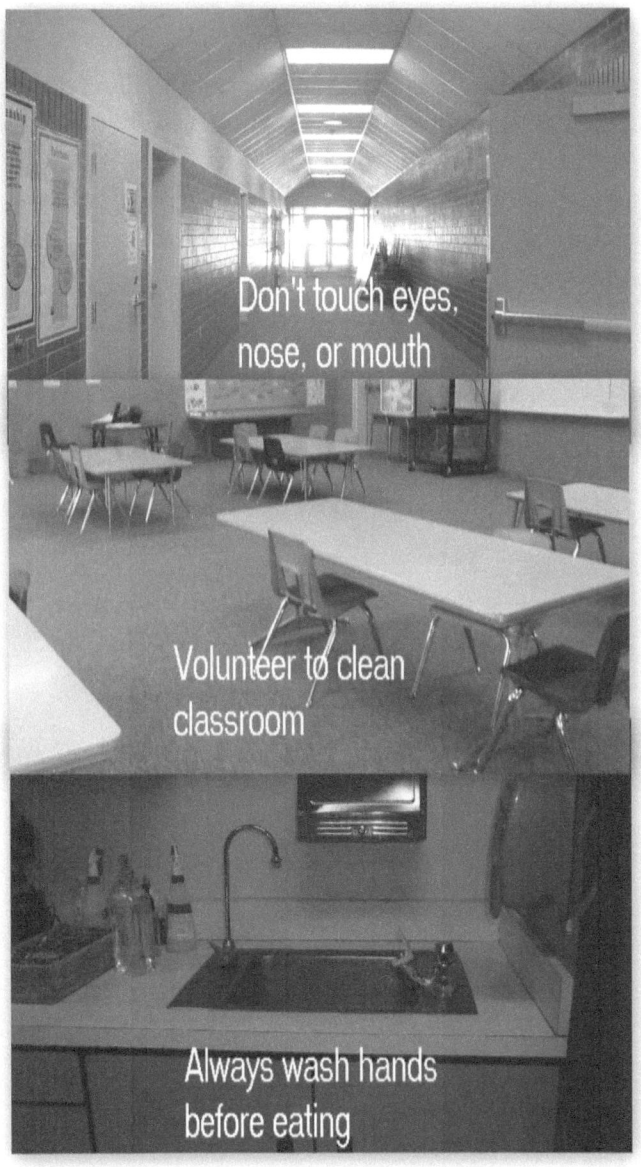

Sports

Locker rooms are a breeding ground for germs, including the dreaded MRSA (methicillin resistant staphylococcus aureus). Never share towels, razors, bar soap, or any items of clothing. Make sure all equipment is thoroughly sanitized after each use. Wash your body thoroughly with liquid soap after every practice and game.

If you are in a contact sport such as wrestling, don't be afraid to ask the other team if they have had any problems with MRSA, hepatitis, or any other communicable diseases.

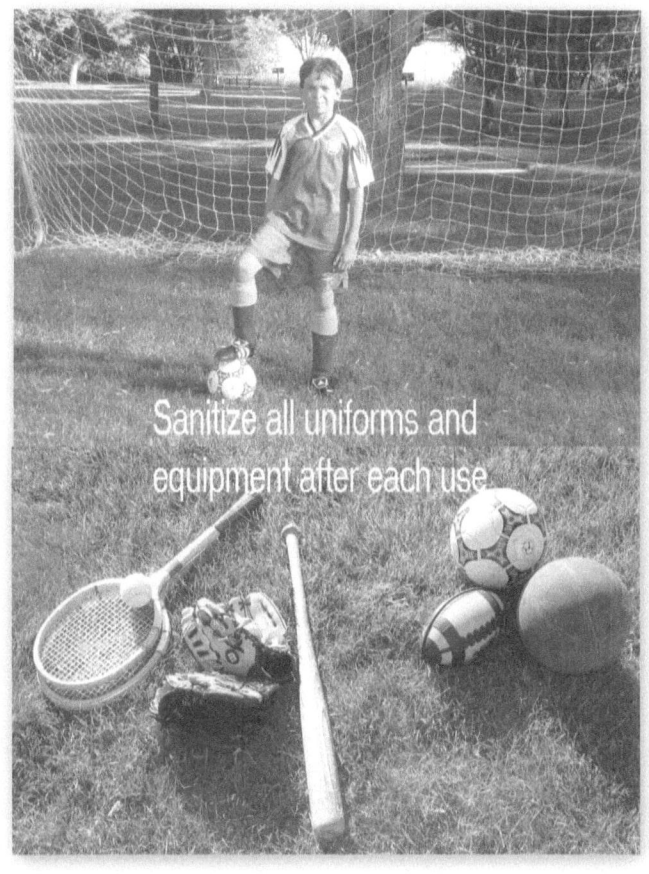

Sanitize all uniforms and
equipment after each use.

GYMS/FITNESS CENTERS

When working out at a public gym, bring your own books and magazines to avoid touching theirs. Wipe the machines off before and after each use. If you are doing floor exercises that require a floor mat, bring your own. Do not use their floor mats! Always shower when you get home and wash your workout clothes and equipment.

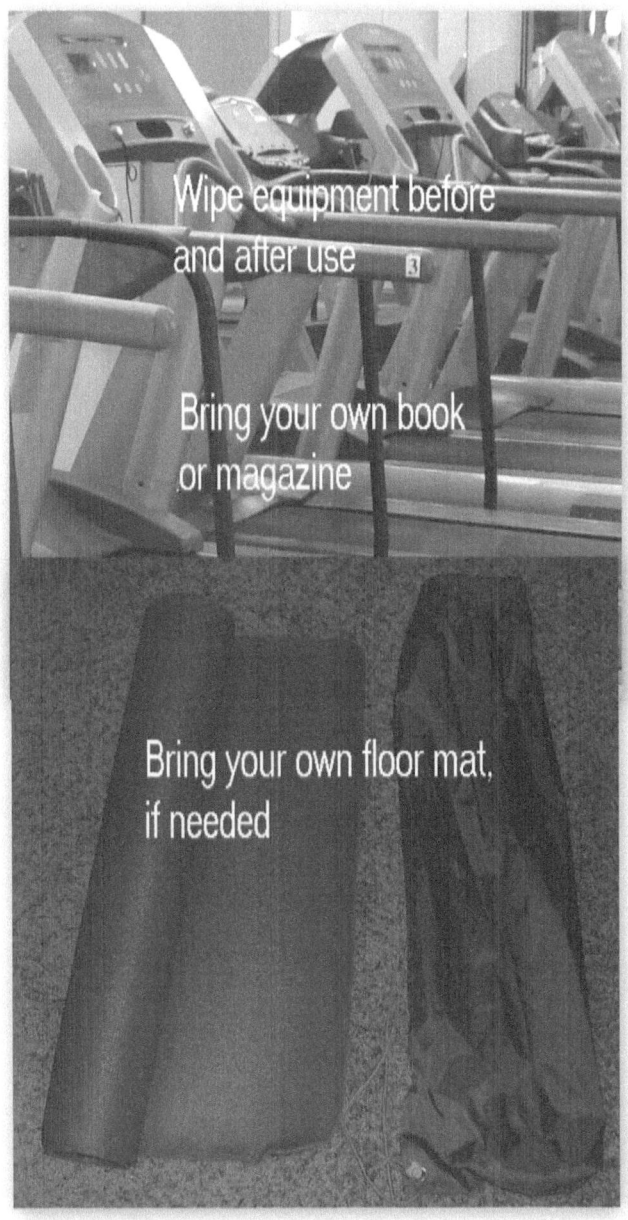

Wipe equipment before
and after use

Bring your own book
or magazine

Bring your own floor mat,
if needed

PUBLIC POOLS

Always wear water shoes at the public pool to avoid getting athlete's foot. If you plan on using one of the lounge chairs around the pool, bring an extra towel to cover it. Watch news reports or newspapers about pools that may have problems with cryptosporidium, which is resistant to the chlorine in the pool and causes severe cramping, vomiting, fever, and diarrhea. If there is a pool in your area that has ultraviolet treatment systems that kill cryptosporidium, choose that pool over one that does not have the UV treatment. Do not swim at all for two weeks if you have had diarrhea to avoid spreading cryptosporidium to other people. Put all diaper aged kids in swim diapers.

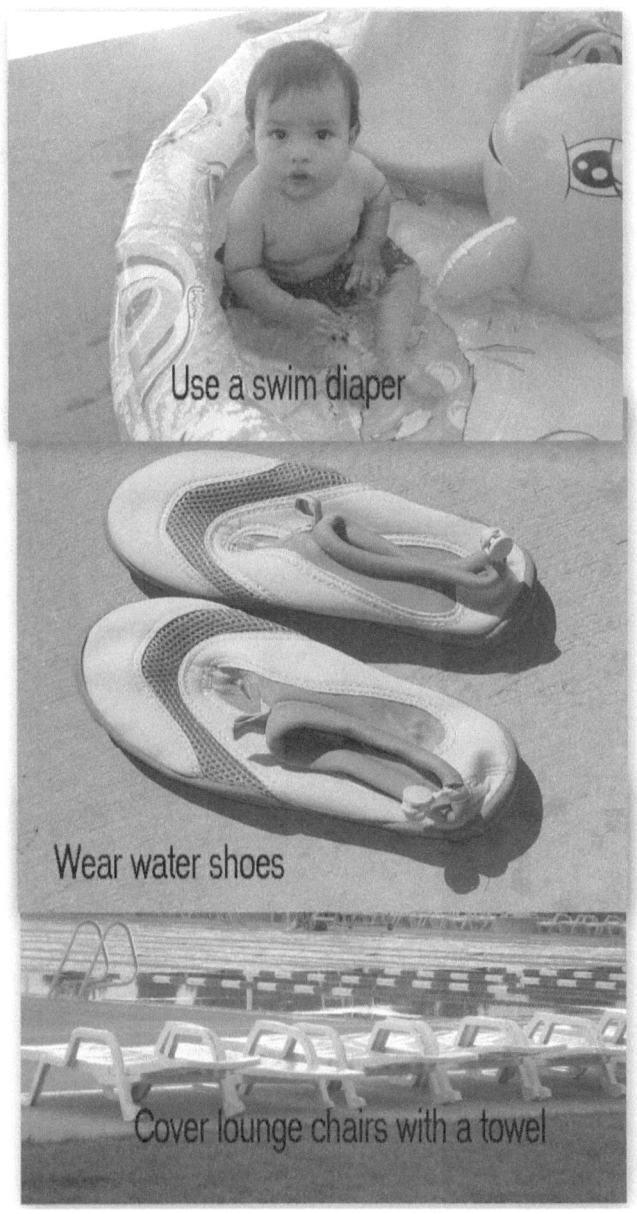

Use a swim diaper

Wear water shoes

Cover lounge chairs with a towel

Public Playgrounds

Since it's not practical to sanitize an entire public playground, teach your children to avoid touching their eyes, nose, and mouth while playing. If you are having a picnic at the park, eat first, then play. Don't give your child suckers or any type of candy when they are running around a public playground since touching the equipment will dirty their hands. Sanitize their hands when they are done playing and give them a bath or shower when you get home.

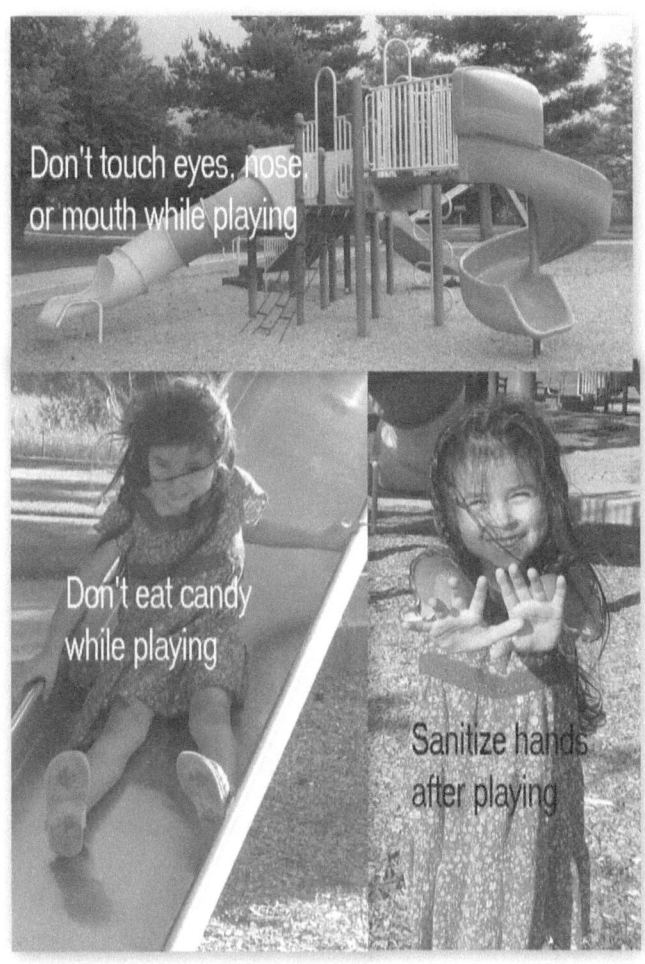

AMUSEMENT PARKS

Like public playgrounds, you can't sanitize all of the rides at an amusement park. Avoid touching your eyes, nose, and mouth. Clean your hands thoroughly before eating anything. Shower and change your clothes when you get home.

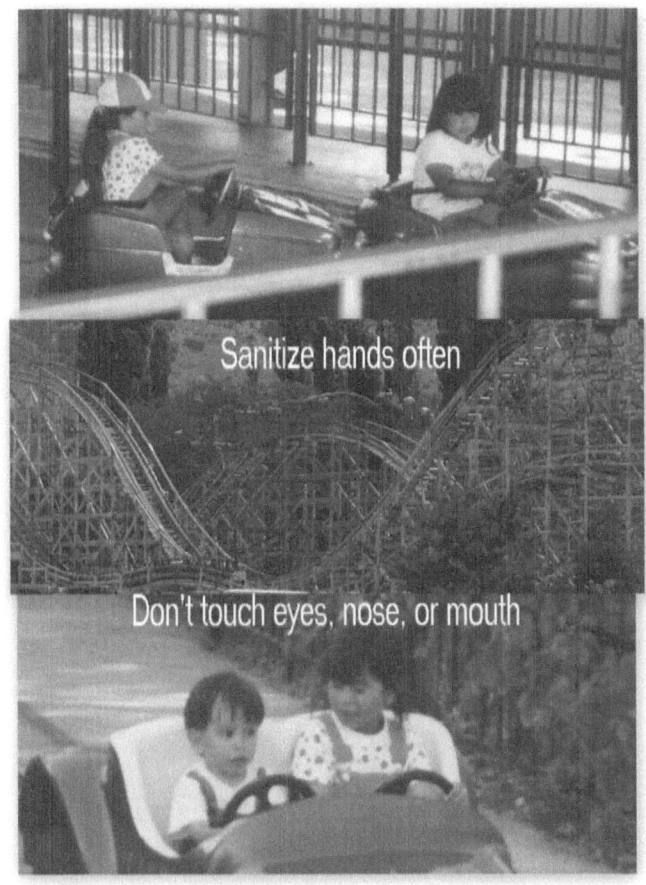

Outdoor Picnic Tables

Outdoor picnic tables have birds, bugs, and possibly animals crawling on them. The best thing to do is cover it. Use a disposable tablecloth, or an old sheet that can be washed with bleach.

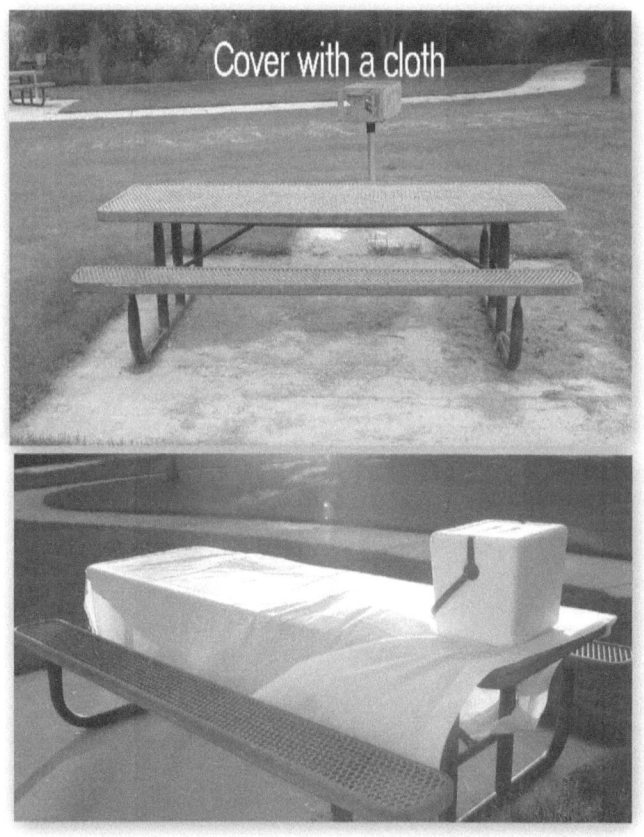

Airports/Airplanes

Airports have travelers from all over the world. They are likely to have germs that you have not been exposed to before, which increases your risk of getting sick. Be extra careful about what you touch and sanitize your hands often. If you rent a cart to carry your luggage, sanitize it like you would a grocery cart.

The inside of an airplane is a confined space and you are stuck there with all of the airborne germs that other passengers may have brought on board with them. Take an immunity-boosting supplement before and after air travel.

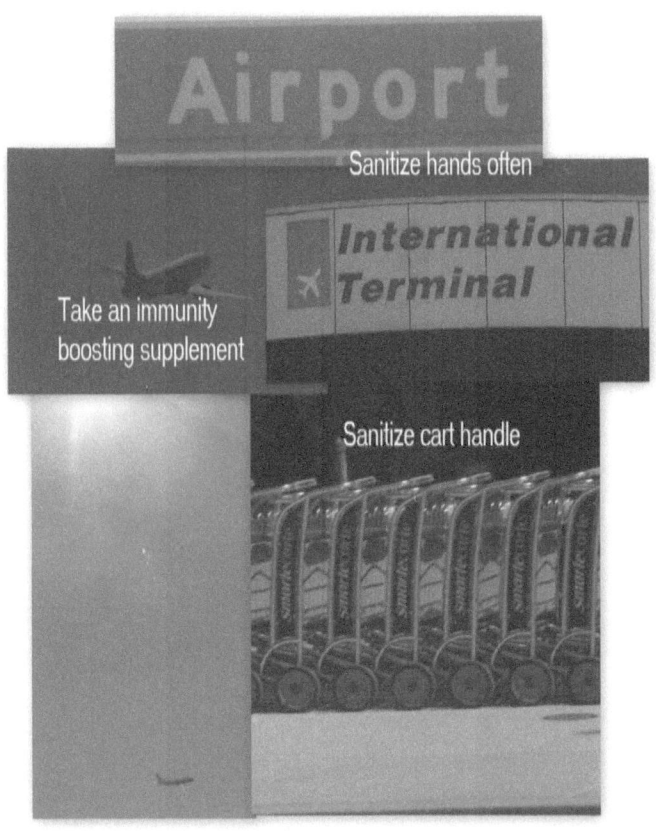

HOTEL/MOTEL ROOMS

When sleeping at a hotel or motel, keep in mind that only the sheets and pillowcases on the beds are washed after each use. Fold the sheet over the blanket and bedspread to avoid touching them. Don't walk around barefoot on the carpet. Spray the upholstered chairs with a sanitizing spray. Disinfect counters with a sanitizing wipe or spray. Most hotels are good about cleaning their rooms, but you just don't know if it has been thoroughly sanitized or just made to look clean.

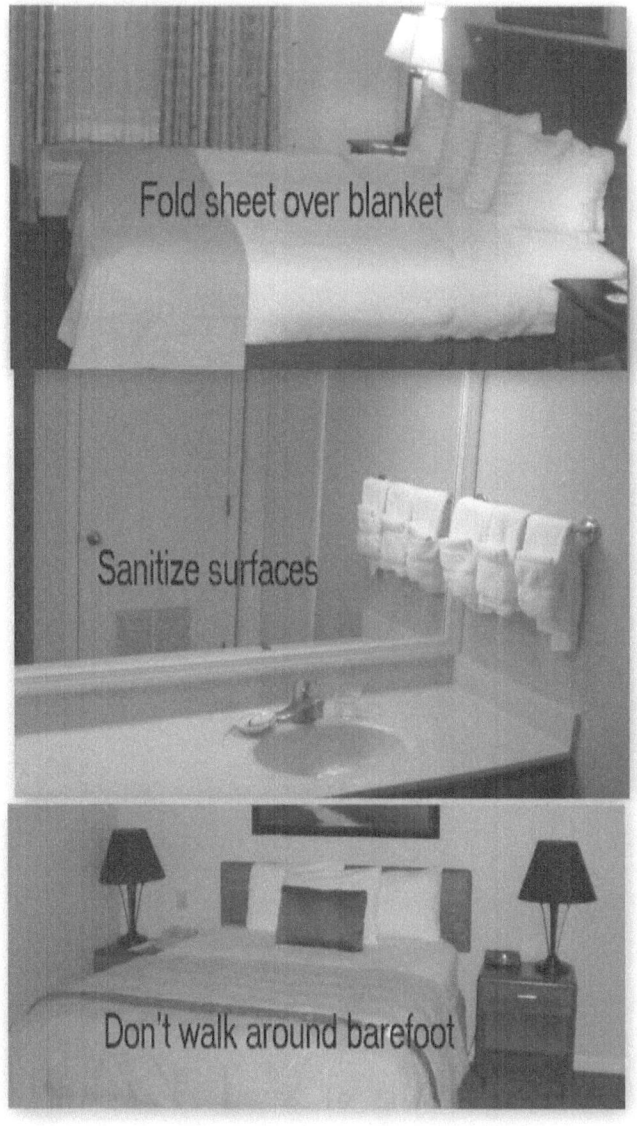

Bar Soap vs. Liquid Soap

Avoid using bar soap. It harbors bacteria. Bar soap will put more germs on you than it removes. Liquid soap is a much better choice both for hand washing, bathing, and showers.

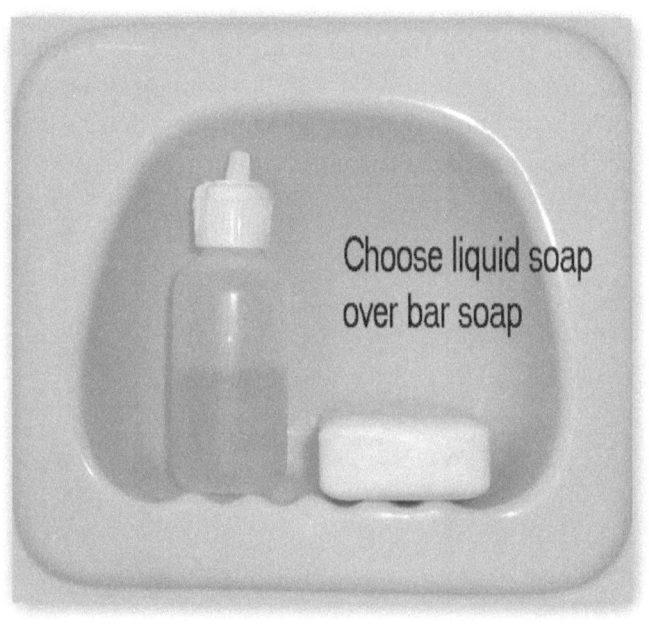

Choose liquid soap over bar soap

DOCTOR'S OFFICE/HOSPITAL

Doctor's office and hospital waiting areas are full of sick people and their germs. Try to find an isolated place to sit. Bring your own magazine or book to read instead of touching theirs. Bring something to entertain your kids as well to prevent them from touching the toys and books that are provided. Be observant of the doctors and nurses hand washing practices. Don't be afraid to ask them to wash their hands if you think it is needed. It is also a good idea to take an immunity-boosting supplement before or after visiting the doctor's office since there are likely to be germs in the air

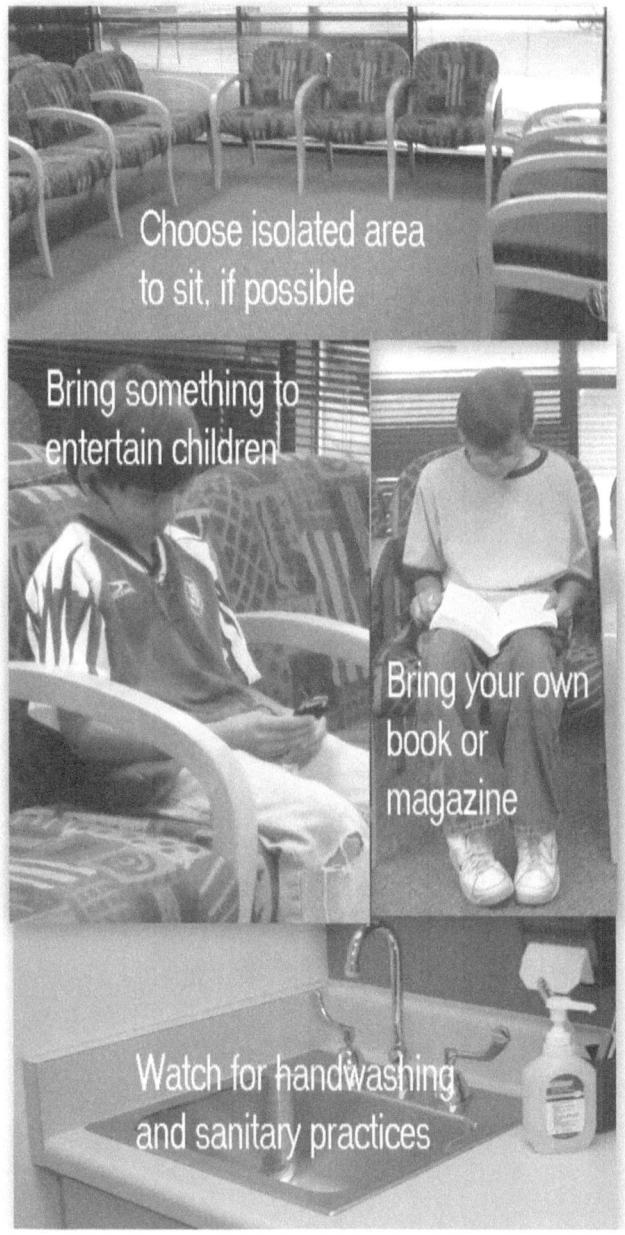

Choose isolated area to sit, if possible

Bring something to entertain children

Bring your own book or magazine

Watch for handwashing and sanitary practices

WHEN YOU GET SICK

It doesn't matter how careful you are, everybody gets sick at some point. Colds in the winter can be especially hard to avoid. Cough into your arm, not on your hands! Stay home to avoid spreading your germs to others. Use a sanitizing spray to kill airborne germs. Sanitize commonly used surfaces such as doorknobs, faucets, light switches and phones daily. Clean bathrooms thoroughly. Wash your sheets and pillowcases when you are feeling better. Disinfect all of the areas that you came into contact with while you were sick.

If you absolutely must go out while you are sick, please be considerate of others and wear a mask.

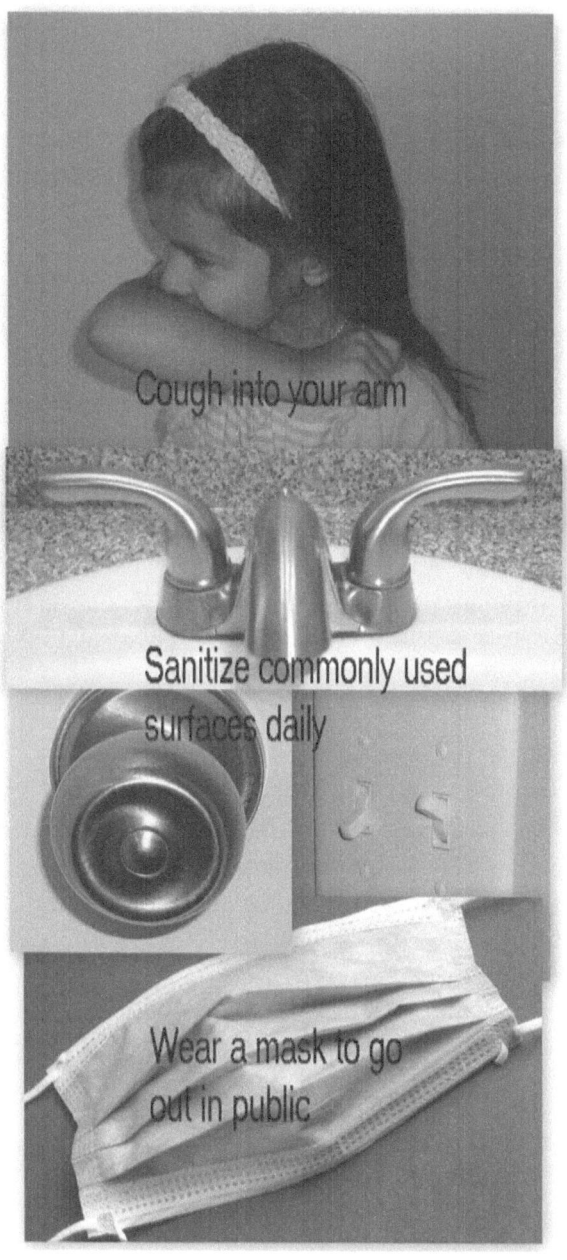

General Household Germophobe Tips

1. Never wipe countertops or tables with a sponge. Use a clean dishcloth.
2. Keep commonly used electronics such as phones, mp3 players, video games, computer keyboards, TV remote controls, etc. clean.
3. Periodically sanitize all children's toys, especially after an illness. Children can help with this chore.
4. Keep light switches, refrigerator handles, faucet handles, sinks, tubs, toilets, countertops, doorknobs, floors, etc. clean.
5. Use specific laundry baskets for clean clothes only. Have separate baskets or hampers for dirty clothes.
6. Always wash your hands after handling dirty clothes.
7. Keep a supply of rubber gloves in the house for cleaning and handling raw meat.
8. Periodically sanitize car door handles and steering wheel.
9. Remove shoes inside the house to avoid spreading dirt and germs on the floors.
10. Periodically sanitize trashcans. Smaller ones can fit in the dishwasher (without dishes of course).